Pilates

Thorsons First Directions

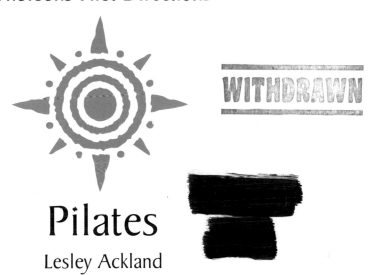

Pilates

Lesley Ackland

Thorsons
An Imprint of HarperCollins*Publishers*
77–85 Fulham Palace Road,
Hammersmith, London W6 8JB

The Thorsons website is: www.thorsons.com

Published by Thorsons 2001

10 9 8 7 6 5 4 3 2 1

Text derived from *Pilates Body Power*, published by Thorsons 2001

Editor: Jillian Stewart
Design: Wheelhouse Creative
Production: Melanie Vandevelde
Photography by Guy Hearn

A catalogue record for this book
is available from the British Library

ISBN 0 00712355 8

Printed and bound in Hong Kong

Contents

Pilates

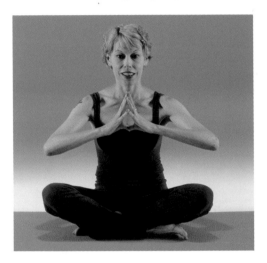

Pilates is a disciplined, focused form of exerci
and joints, increase flexibility and lengthen th

signed to strengthen ligaments
uscles

Introduction

Do you dream of a flat stomach, a longer, leaner body and superb posture? Do you wish to improve your overall appearance? If so, then Pilates will help you achieve all this – and more. In this book you will discover a unique bodywork system that will help you transform your body and develop a physical presence and energy that exudes total confidence and grace.

While most people have heard of Pilates, few know exactly what it entails. Pilates is a very disciplined, focused form of exercise, designed to strengthen ligaments and joints, increase flexibility and lengthen the muscles. The main emphasis is on 'elongating' the body to create a longer, leaner and taller silhouette. However, Pilates differs from other exercise regimes by going beyond the purely physical. This is a holistic discipline that integrates the mind, body and spirit. It is a philosophy of movement that brings about mental and physical integration.

If you have never tried this type of exercise before, you will be surprised by its apparent simplicity. The slow, controlled movements enable energy to move more freely throughout the body. The visualization techniques gently help to focus the mind so that each exercise is executed with ultimate precision. With Pilates there is no need for over-exertion. The emphasis is on quality, not quantity. It's not about how much you do but, rather, how you do it. This is good news indeed for those of you who have become disillusioned and bored with fitness programmes that may not suit you.

If you want a long, lean look, with a minimum of effort in the safest way, you merely have to follow the guidelines in this book. Most of the techniques are based on the idea of using your own body to create resistance, so there is no need for any complicated props. All you need is a willing body and a curious mind. Before you attempt any of the exercises though, it is important that you first become acquainted with the underlying principles outlined in chapters one to four.

Pilates promises no quick fixes or sudden improvements. However, with concentration and commitment, the end result will be rewarding and nothing short of enhanced physical and mental well-being.

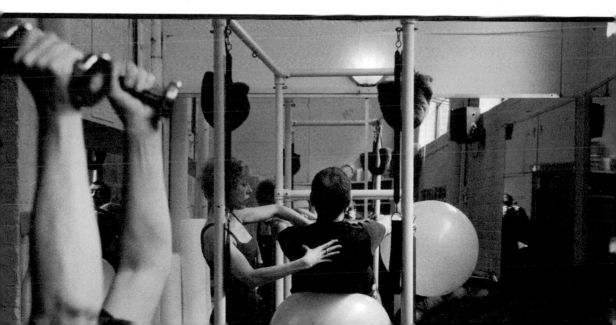

The origins of classic pilates

The original concept of Pilates was the brainchild of a German, Josef Hubertus Pilates. He was extremely frail and weak as a child, but was determined to regain good health. This was the start of a life-long obsession with fitness and body building, and as a young man he excelled as a diver, skier and professional gymnast. Aged 32 he decided to move to England, where he made a living as a boxer, circus performer and self-defence instructor.

When the First World War broke out, his career was temporarily cut short. As a German, Pilates was interned in England for the duration of the war. He used this time, however, as an opportunity to re-think and develop his approach to fitness. The result was the first blueprint for a whole new regime, Pilates, which drew upon all the various disciplines with which he was involved. His basic philosophy concluded that the only way to achieve true fitness was through the integration of mind and body. Hence, all his techniques were based on a combination of physical and mental conditioning.

When Josef Pilates created his unique system of exercise during the early part of the twentieth century the lifestyle was, in many respects, healthier for the public at large. People walked far more, for instance, and were not subject to the repetitive movements inherent in using a computer or sitting in an office chair all day. For this reason I decided to expand and enhance the basic principles of Pilates.

Body maintenance

In 1980 I began developing Body Maintenance, a balanced system of exercise, body shaping and tone combined with mental improvement and nutrition, based on Pilates. This unique bodywork system integrates methods from a wide variety of sources, including remedial massage, osteopathy and injury clinics. In my studio in London's Covent Garden I use the system to treat people suffering from modern infirmities such as RSI, as well as giving classes for those whose focus is simply on gaining or maintaining fitness.

   The Pilates-based exercises I teach in my studio often incorporate balls, ropes, springs and pulleys. However, the most important and long-lasting work takes place on the floor. Mat exercises, essential to body mobility and endurance, target weak, under-utilized muscles in the abdomen, lower back, arms and legs. The exercises in this book are based on mat work. They involve straightforward, concentrated movements that don't require a gym or special equipment. What they do require is a little time, be it in the morning, during lunch time or later in the evening. This is a complete exercise regime devised for individuals who might not have the inclination or opportunity to seek out my studio, but who want to benefit from my tried and proven Pilates-based exercise programme.

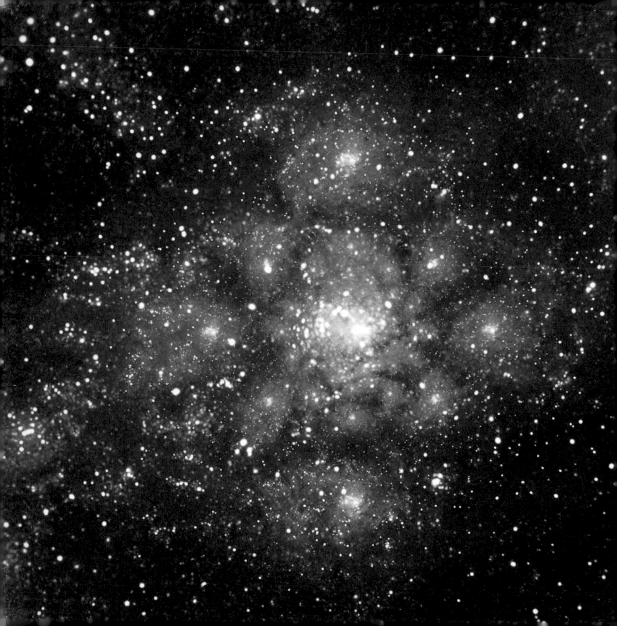

The Mind-body Connection

The main principle of Pilates is that exercise is essentially a mind–body technique. Therefore, when you exercise you mentally focus on the muscle groups that you are using. Pilates recognizes that it is only through the synchronizing of thought and action that an exercise is truly effective. In order to create a healthy and fit body you need to integrate the mental, physical and spiritual spheres.

Mind over matter

It has long been established that the mind has an enormous influence on the health of the body. Research shows that the mind has an infinite capacity to induce positive physiological effects. You may have noticed that when you're in a good mood you automatically seem to look and feel better. Scientists ascribe this phenomenon to the activity of the billions of nerve cells in our brain, which transmit chemical messages to the rest of the body. Our thoughts and emotions play a vital role in influencing this intercellular communication.

Think for a moment how you feel when you are stressed. Not very pleasant. This is because your body produces an excess of 'stress' chemicals (e.g., adrenaline and cortisol), which causes your whole system to speed up. Your heart beats faster, your blood pressure goes up, your breathing becomes rapid and shallow. At times, this type of response is necessary. It is what motivates you when you are faced with a crisis. In large doses this type of reaction can, however, be extremely harmful and lead to all sorts of unpleasant symptoms such as dizziness, profuse sweating, insomnia and migraines. In contrast, positive feelings of calm and contentment have a much more beneficial effect, as they induce the body to produce health enhancing, 'feel-good' chemicals (e.g., endorphins and serotonin), which are vital for well-being. They promote a sense of serenity – you breathe more easily and deeply, your heart rate is slower and your blood pressure lowers. The more relaxed you feel, the less tension you hold in the muscles throughout your body. This has a beneficial effect on your general bearing and posture. Tight, tense muscles make your body shrink and constrict. This stops the energy from flowing freely throughout the body and, in time, this will be reflected in a weak, misshapen musculature.

Mindful exercise

If thoughts are so powerful, it makes sense to try and harness your thinking to bring about positive changes in your body. This is, in fact, the very essence of Pilates. By learning to execute each exercise correctly you are also allowing your mind to exert a greater influence over your body. With Pilates you only do a limited number of repetitions. You do them slowly, so that you can concentrate more clearly on directing your energy towards what it is that you are trying to achieve. If you view your body in a negative way you will need to reverse your direction of thought. Positive thoughts bring about positive changes.

To ensure that an exercise can be of real benefit and will bring about the changes that you desire, for example a strong, straight back, it is necessary to complement each physical action with a mental focus. Painting a picture in your mind of what you want to achieve helps your body to respond in the right way. By practising creative visualization regularly, you will gradually develop the intellectual and emotional ability to internalize the physical changes that you wish to make. Once you've done this, the external changes will start to appear.

Creative visualization

Whatever we create in our lives begins as a basic image in our minds. Many of these images are unconscious. Through creative visualization it is possible to alter these thoughts and pictures. With Pilates, the idea is to create an image in your mind that will help you to focus on the area of the body that you are working. This requires a very deep level of concentration, which does become easier with practice. On a superficial level, many of the exercises appear quite simple. How you physically position your arms and legs, however, is only part of the process. Pilates, unlike many other disciplines, is actually much more complex, as with each movement you must be constantly aware of what your entire body is doing. You don't concentrate only on the stomach, or the inner thigh, and exclude the rest of your body. Even when you are doing a series of movements specifically designed to work a certain group of muscles, such as your abdominals, you must always remember to be equally focused on the rest of your body. Where are your feet? Are you holding your head in exactly the right way? Is your body properly aligned?

Initially, this can seem quite difficult and using visualization techniques can be enormously helpful. By understanding how your body should be feeling it becomes easier to assume the correct position. Eventually, these images will arise naturally through association, without too much effort.

Basic visualization techniques

Anyone can learn to visualize. It helps though if you can begin by feeling relaxed. A still mind is more conducive to conjuring up images.

- Spend a few minutes gathering your thoughts. Try to forget about external influences such as work. Remember, this is your time.
- Do some gentle stretches and focus on your breathing. Slow, deep breathing has an instantly calming effect. Once you are feeling sufficiently relaxed you can start your exercises.
- As you exercise, focus on each part of your body. How does it feel? With each exercise try to perceive a specific picture. If you are trying to see yourself on a sandy beach, focus clearly on how this feels. Do your feet feel relaxed? Are your arms hanging loosely by your sides? Think of images that will help you to get into exactly the right position.
- Invite each image to emerge with as much intensity as possible, so that you can almost feel it. Once you have created a familiar picture, eventually all you will have to do is focus on it and your body will automatically respond.

The aim of Pilates is to bring about permanent changes. You can hasten this process by using visualization techniques when you are not exercising. These will automatically help you to walk, stand and sit in the correct way.

Essentials

Pilates is a very precise system of exercise. It is different from other regimes in that it requires a bit of groundwork before you start. In order to understand fully what you are doing it is important that you first become acquainted with the basic principles. There are six essential guidelines to remember.

1. Breathing

Pilates differs from conventional forms of exercise in that it concentrates on the correct use of breathing for each and every exercise. Breath nourishes the body and the brain. People tend to breathe shallowly into their upper bodies when they inhale, into the upper chest and not right down into their lower lobes. If you are breathing deeply, you're working from the inside out. You are energizing and replenishing large areas of your body. It is as much a spiritual as a physical idea.

For most of the exercises in this book, you will breathe out on the point of effort. During the exercises think about oxygen as a rejuvenating life-force. Always exhale on the point of effort. If you have a tight area, try and breathe into that – breath is another form of liberation, working from the inside out.

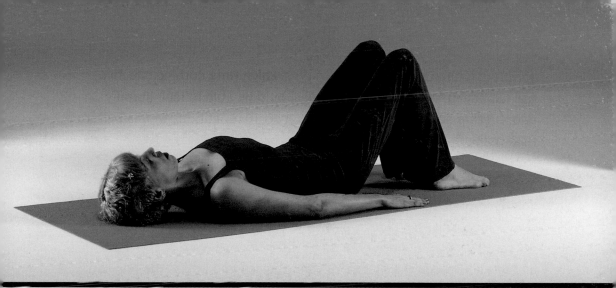

2. Control

All the exercises in Pilates are controlled. In this particular instance the word 'controlled' means that the correct body parts are being used. Many people, for example, thinking that they are using their abdominals during an exercise, are, in fact using their bones or hip flexors. Thus, the muscles that should be targeted are not being worked in an efficient way.

Control and precision go together. All these exercises are done slowly, in a meditative fashion. You focus the mind on what you're doing, and don't allow it to wander. You use breath, coordination, control and precision to do a limited number of repetitions well.

You minimize the stress and involvement of other parts of the body. It's preferable to do even five repetitions in a slow and regulated way, than to go through hundreds of motions, during which time nothing effective has happened. In the pelvic tilts, you should be able to feel, literally, one vertebra at a time. The fact that you do 10 repetitions well is better than doing many repetitions badly.

3. Centring

The main principle of the Pilates technique is to recognize that there is one strong, core area that controls the rest of the body. This is located in that part of your body which forms a continuous band at the back and front, between the bottom of your rib-cage and across the line of your hipbones. This is called the centre. This is the area in which the muscles in your stomach and back are – at the centre of your body. These muscles support the internal organs and keep you upright. If you have a strong centre you have a strong back, which means you can walk, stand and run without discomfort or pain. Your arms and legs are extensions of this part of your body. If you have a bad back this is an indication that the centre is not strong enough. Originally human beings were not designed to stand upright. The only reason we stand at all is due to these specific muscles.

We are constantly fighting gravity, which pulls us forward. This explains why so many people have all sorts of problems with those muscles affiliated with the shoulders and neck. We are basically defying nature, gravity and our initial body type.

4. Flow

Each movement in Pilates is designed to be performed in a smooth, flowing, undulating way. There is no room within this regime for any sharp, jarring movements or quick, jerky actions – these are the total antithesis of everything you are trying to achieve. If a movement ever feels like this, you can be sure that you are doing it wrong. Every motion originates from a strong centre and flows in a slow, gentle, controlled fashion. This warms the muscles, causing them to lengthen and open up the spaces between each vertebra in the spine so that the body expands to create a longer, leaner shape.

5. Precision

In order to be effective, all Pilates exercises have to be performed with exact precision. This attention to detail is important as it ensures that each movement is working the body in the correct manner. Before you start an exercise sequence, read the instructions carefully. Pay full attention to proper alignment and check what the 'watchpoints' have to say. This will ensure that you do not expend excess energy doing an exercise incorrectly.

6. Coordination

Children run naturally, but for most adults basic coordination is a major problem. Many people, when starting these exercises, complain to me, 'I can't coordinate my breath and the movement. It's too much. I've got to concentrate too hard. I can't do it.' Most of us have lost the ability to coordinate the mind and body into a working machine. We no longer have the sense of our feet being in contact with the earth. We've lost the feeling of the way the breath moves naturally through the body. The aim is to retrain the neuromuscular connection between the brain and the body.

This is best illustrated when I try and teach foot exercises to people. I sometimes joke that the feet are very far from the brain and they won't obey, as they haven't been asked to do anything for a long time. Observe people who have lost the use of their hands. They can do the same things with their feet that we can do with our hands. We all have that capability, but we don't employ it. If you don't avail yourself of something it atrophies. Therefore, if you don't use coordination in the physical sense you lose the ability. In Pilates, we try to re-create your body as a coordinated whole, rather than thinking 'I am exercising an arm or leg or the stomach.' Coordination is paramount to the way the exercises flow.

Key terms

In Pilates there are certain key terms that are referred to over and over again. It helps if you understand these before you begin. Also take note of the specific guidance on the feet and the neck.

Relaxing

Pilates frequently refers to keeping an area relaxed. This isn't necessarily what you might think. Most people associate relaxation with a feeling of 'letting go', of allowing muscles to slump. In this case, to relax means to release tension in an area while still managing to maintain tone and control. This should feel comfortable and natural.

Neutral spine

Some of the positions you will be assuming require your spine to remain in neutral. This means that you maintain the natural curve in your back. Thus, when you are lying down, do not press your back so hard into the floor that you lose your natural curve. Neither must you allow your back to arch so that your lower back comes off the floor. Just lie there, breathe in and out naturally and allow your back to relax into the floor without pressing it in. This will permit your back to relax into its natural, neutral position – which is slightly different for everybody.

The centre

Each of the exercises originates from the centre. The stomach muscles are the core to everything and support the spine. It is important that you always remember to keep this area correctly aligned. This is particularly important when you exercise the lower abdominals as it is very easy to do the opposite of what you actually want. It is natural when you breathe in for the stomach to pull into the spine and when you breathe out for it to bulge. This is not what you want. You will have to try and reverse what the body wants to do unconsciously. As you breathe in you should relax the stomach; as you breathe out you should pull the navel to the spine, engaging the lower abdominal muscles. Your body will naturally want to do the opposite, but it's important to engage the stomach muscles when you exhale.

One vertebra at a time

Pilates frequently refers to the term one vertebra at a time. This is one of the main principles that you should keep in mind whenever you are doing an exercise that involves rolling your body up from and down to the mat. The idea is that you always roll up gradually so that you are lifting only one vertebra off the mat at a time. The same rule applies when you roll back down again. This takes some practice and initially you will need to concentrate very carefully to ensure that you are doing it correctly.

Straight arms and legs

This is a very common term in Pilates. Your arms and legs should be relaxed and not locked. This is an important point to remember, particularly for the stretches. If an exercise requires that you stretch your arm or leg out straight, you should take care not to overextend, which causes the joints to lock.

The feet

The main thing to remember when exercising is that most of the time you want your feet to be relaxed. If you are in doubt – relax your feet. Most people tense their feet too much and as a result constantly complain about getting cramp in their feet when they are exercising. (If you do get cramp use a foot roller to ease away the tension.) A relaxed foot should feel comfortable, so that there is no sensation of tightness. Whenever you are required to flex your feet, do so by gently stretching out your heel then pulling the top of your foot as far as you can without straining. Do not tense your foot so that it feels strained.

The neck

This is a sensitive part of the body, so you do not want to put it under unnecessary strain while you are exercising. It is very important that you always follow the neck instructions very carefully. Pilates often refers to keeping your neck long, which means adjusting your head into a position that lengthens your neck. When you are doing an exercise lying on your back, the way you bring your head into alignment with the rest of your body is by moving the top of your skull and the base of your neck. Do not attempt to flatten your neck against the floor.

Preparation

The Pilates-based Body Maintenance exercises require total concentration and focus. This makes it particularly important to find a time and place to do them where you know you will not be disturbed. It helps if you get into the right frame of mind. Do this by thinking – this is my time, I am creating a space within my house, within my environment, to work on my body for myself, without distractions.

When to exercise

The exercises can be done at any time of day. You might find you prefer to do them in the early evening, to help you unwind and loosen tight muscles after a busy day. If you find it difficult to get going in the mornings, a 15-minute session first thing may be just what you need.

Clothes

Ideally, you should wear clothing in which you can exercise comfortably, such as leggings, shorts and a T-shirt, or leotard top. Don't wear anything which will restrict your movements. Opt for natural fibres like cotton, which are cooler. You can exercise wearing socks or in bare feet. If you are concerned about slipping, put on a pair of trainers. Take off any jewellery which might get in the way.

Equipment

Most of the exercises require little or no equipment. It is essential however to work on a padded surface or a mat. This will protect your spine and prevent any bruising against a hard floor. It is probably worth investing in a proper sports mat. Alternatively, you can work on a folded, synthetic blanket. This should be about five or six feet long and a foot wide. Ankle weights are used in some of the exercises but this is optional. If an exercise indicates that you need a couple of light handweights and you don't have any, you can substitute cans of beans. If possible, try exercising in front of a full-length mirror. This will enable you to check what you are doing.

Which exercises?

Begin with the posture and balance exercises. The programme then really gets underway with the pelvic tilts and abdominal exercises. It is really important to always do the pelvic tilts and the abdominal exercises before working on the other areas of the body, as this tones

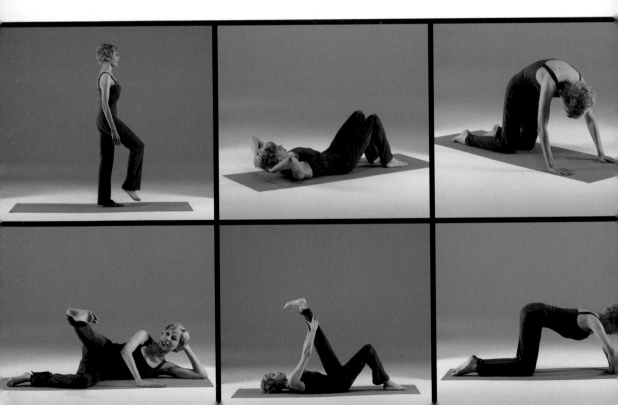

the area and enables you to work from a strong centre. Even when working your arms and legs everything is controlled from the centre. As well as doing some basic abdominal work, each session you do should also incorporate stretches after the relevant strengthening exercises. You can then do upper and lower body work on alternate days.

Sequence of exercises

Warm up with the posture and balance exercises.
1)   Do all the pelvic tilt and abdominal exercises first.
2)   Proceed to the back exercises.
3)   Do leg exercises and stretches.
4)   Finish with upper body exercises and stretches.

Read all the instructions carefully. Remember the breathing instructions.

Continue to add exercises each day as you feel more comfortable. Use your own judgement. If you are unsure do the pelvic tilts and abdominal exercises, then add to them. If you feel any discomfort in your back during any particular exercise, you still have insufficient core strength to do it.

In Pilates-based Body Maintenance there are a number of basic safety rules:

- Always do stretches after the relevant strengthening exercises.
- Do not attempt to do too much too soon. Increase the number of repetitions gradually.
- If you feel nauseous, fatigued or extremely breathless – stop.
- If you have any chest pains (especially when accompanied by pain in the arm, neck, shoulders and jaw) – stop exercising immediately and seek medical help.
- If exercise leaves you unnaturally tired, check with your doctor.
- The neck is a sensitive area of the body. If you cannot remember whether you have worked this area or not, it is better not to do any further repetitions.
- Always make sure that there is something you can hold on to for support when doing the balancing exercises.
- If you experience back pain – stop.
- If your muscles start shaking – stop.
- Drink plenty of fluids afterwards, especially when it is hot.

Before you embark on any new programme, it's a good idea to consult your doctor. A pre-exercise check-up is strongly advised if you are over 40 or have not been exercising regularly. Always seek the advice of a specialist if you have a medical condition, are pregnant or have any chronic joint problems.

The Exercise Programme

The exercises in this programme will help you to tone and strengthen specific muscles in your stomach, back, legs, chest and arms. In time, as your body adapts, you will also start to look taller, slimmer and more youthful.

Before you attempt any of the exercises in the rest of the chapter, start with the following essential posture and balance exercises. It is best to do these in bare feet. If you've got a mirror – even better. That way, you'll be able to keep an eye on what you're doing and make sure that it's correct. If you lack good posture and balance, practise these exercises every day.

Perfect posture

Stand with your feet hip-width apart. Imagine that you're standing on sand. Your feet are relaxed. Think of your weight being over the middle of each foot, with your toes gently lengthening into the sand. Close your eyes and make a mental note of the following:

- Don't sink back into your heels or lean forward. Keep your weight evenly distributed over your feet.
- Let your arms fall naturally in front of your body.
- Let your hands hang from the shoulders, totally loose and relaxed.
- Don't lock your knees. They should feel relaxed and not rigid.
- Keep your inside thighs and bottom relaxed.
- Imagine that your head is like one of those nodding dogs in the back of car. It's not going backwards and forwards but resting directly upon your shoulders and rocking gently until it settles into a comfortable, neutral position.
- Think of the bones directly behind your ears. Try to imagine them 'reaching' towards the ceiling.
- Pull your stomach in, without tipping the pelvis forward. Think of a piece of string from your pubic bone to your navel. It is shortening as you pull up and in. Feel your tailbone drop – as if it is weighted to the floor.
- Keep the front of your thighs relaxed.

Now your whole body is perfectly aligned – you should feel as if you are floating an inch off the ground.

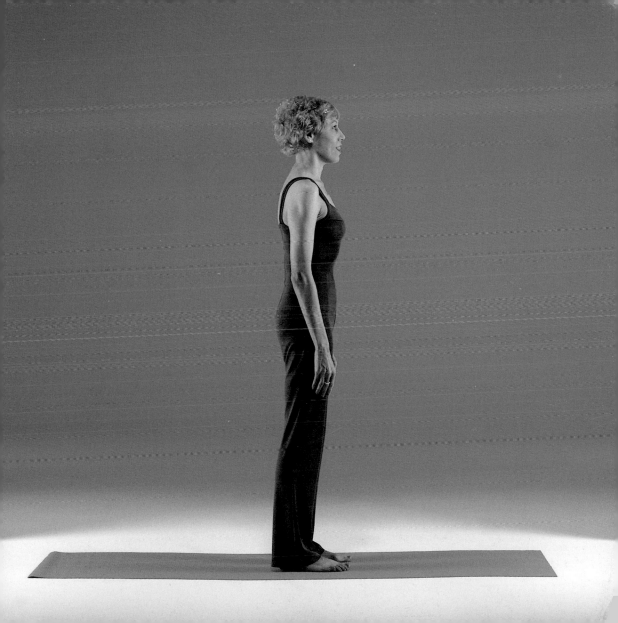

Exercises for better balance

If you have a tendency to slip or trip and are unable to catch objects thrown towards you, your sense of balance is probably poor. What seems to occur, as you get older or as a result of injury, is that you lose your awareness of balance and your reflexes are no longer as sharp. This can cause feelings of insecurity. We all know that the simplest of falls might have serious consequences. This is reflected in the body, which becomes stiff and constricted as a result. The following three exercises will, in time, allow you to feel lighter and more confident in the way you move. For each of these exercises all the same rules as the 'perfect posture' exercise apply (*see page* 26).

Walking backwards

Start in the 'perfect posture' position and, with feet approximately an inch apart, start to walk backwards. Slowly drag your foot back, so that it never entirely leaves the floor. The easiest way to master this is to imagine that you are trying to remove some chewing gum from under your feet. Look in the mirror – but do not look down at your feet.

Standing on one leg

With bare feet, stand on one leg, and imagine you are on a beach with soft sand between your toes. Keep your other leg slightly lifted. Count for 10 seconds and change legs. Repeat four times, twice on each leg. Now do the same – with your eyes closed. Make sure you have something to hold onto, lest you fall over.

Standing on one leg on a towel

Do exactly the same as in the previous exercise, standing on a flat towel. This gives you a slightly more unstable surface and makes the exercise more difficult. Even if you don't regularly exercise, try to do these every day – especially if you're over 45.

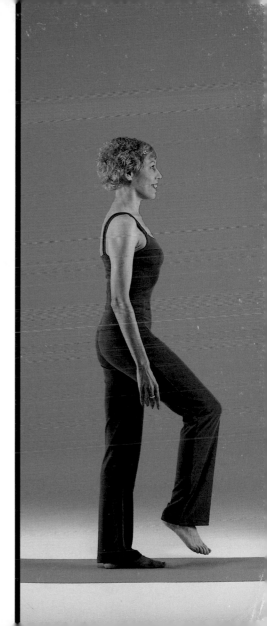

Sitting properly

Generally people sit badly, so this exercise is particularly important for those who sit at a desk or in front of a computer all day. The emphasis here is not on complicated movement but on visualization.

Sit with your back supported by a chair. Your tailbone is heavy, both feet are evenly placed on the floor. You are in contact from your centre directly down through your feet into the floor. Channel your energies from your centre out through the crown of your head. Your shoulders are relaxed, your arms are relaxed because your middle back is supported. Your tailbone will drop and your abdominals will naturally pull back towards your spine. Try to think of your head sitting naturally on top of your shoulders, not pushing forward and not pushing back.

Watchpoint

• Don't force your shoulders back as this will cause your lower back to arch away from the chair.

Breathing

Correct breathing is a very important facet of Pilates. By remembering to breathe properly, you'll find it becomes much easier to exercise. The problem is that most people don't breathe deeply enough. Breathing slowly and deeply is very energizing. It ensures there is sufficient oxygen circulating throughout the body.

It may sound obvious, but when you exercise do not hold your breath. It's better to breathe incorrectly than not at all. Practise the following exercise before you start any of the stomach work.

Basic breathing exercise

- Lie on your back in a relaxed position, resting your head on a folded towel, with your knees bent.
- Place one hand on your stomach and, very gently, breathe in through your nose. Feel your lungs filling with oxygen and slowly expand and relax your stomach. Breathe out.
- With one finger on your pubic bone and one on your navel, try and shorten that gap as you breathe out, and flatten your stomach to your spine without tilting your pelvis.
- Breathe in again and feel that gap slightly expand.
- Breathe out. Imagine there is a piece of string or an elastic band that links your pubic bone to your navel. Very gently feel it pulling up and in. This will get all three sets of stomach muscles working, which will tighten your waist.

Make sure you breathe slowly and deeply. One of the main rules of Pilates is to breathe out on the point of effort. If in doubt, particularly on the stretches, breathe naturally.

When you breathe in your stomach gently expands. However, it shouldn't swell in an exaggerated way. Try and think of your ribcage expanding gently to the sides so that you're not just breathing into your throat and upper chest.

When you begin this exercise programme and you start to breathe properly you might feel a bit dizzy. As you are learning to breathe more deeply, you are taking in more oxygen – which can make you feel a little light-headed.

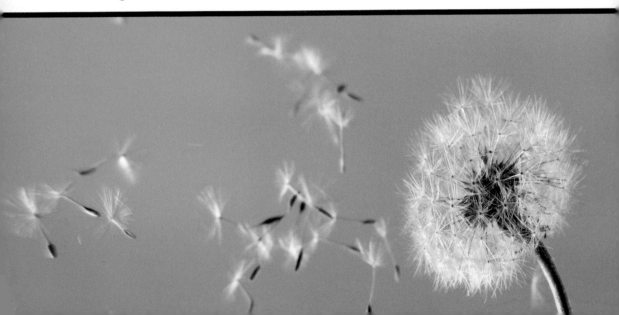

Basic abdominal and back exercises

These basic abdominal and back exercises are good for conditioning, toning and strengthening. In Pilates when you do abdominal work, as you breathe in the stomach gently expands. As you breathe out the stomach pulls in, navel to spine. Feel the connection from the pubic bone up to the navel. The body will automatically want to do the opposite as you breathe out on the point of effort. You inhale through the nose and exhale through the mouth. As you breathe out think about pulling the navel to the spine without tipping the pelvis.

It's better to do these exercises either lying on a towel or on an exercise mat. As you're lying on your back, you may want to place a folded towel under your head. This will help lengthen your neck. If you're not sure about this, try it with and without a small folded towel and see which is more comfortable.

Repeat each exercise 10 times. Do the stretches in sets of four.

Pelvic tilt

The pelvic tilt is a preparation exercise that warms up the back. It's a good starting point, whatever part of the programme you plan to do.

Lie on your back, with your knees bent and parallel, about hip-width apart. Arms should be resting at your sides, with palms facing the floor. This helps to lengthen your neck. Breathe in, then breathe out and gently relax your back into the floor. When you do this, do not press your back too strongly to the ground so that you lose your natural curve. Do not allow your back to arch to the point that it lifts off the floor. This is called the neutral spine position and it is slightly different for everybody (*see page* 17). There is no point in trying to force your back down. Try very hard not to tense your buttock muscles during this exercise.

As you breathe out gently tilt your pelvis forward and roll your lower back off the floor – one vertebra at a time, as you 'peel' your back off the mat (*see page* 18). Breathe in, keeping your neck long, and very slowly roll all the way down, breathing out. Keep your feet relaxed on the floor and imagine that your toes are 'lengthening' away.

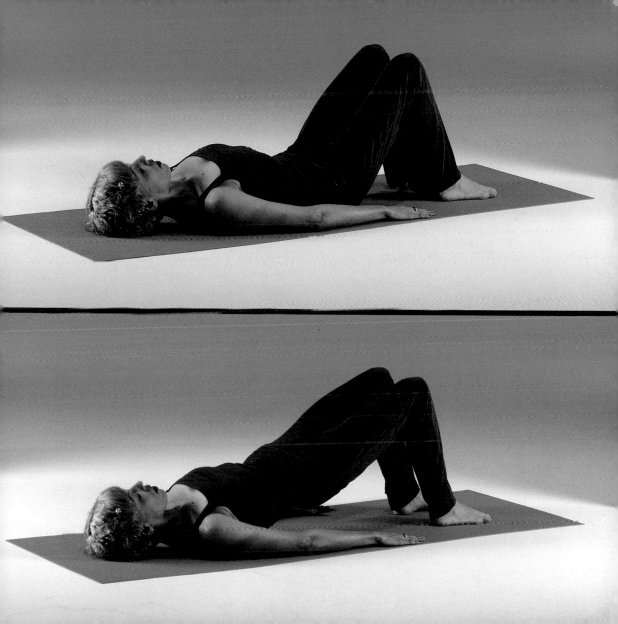

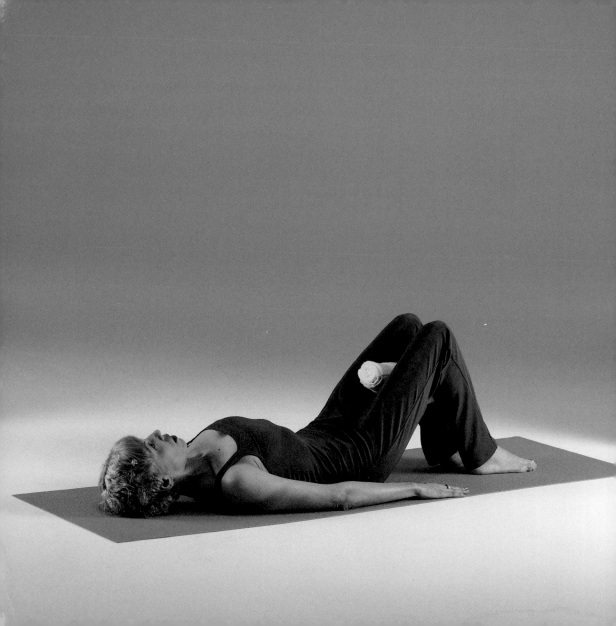

Preparation for abdominals

This is a preparation for the abdominal exercises. It will wake up your stomach muscles and prepare you for the more difficult exercises.

Lie as before – with a relaxed back and long neck, without tucking the pelvis under. Take either a small cushion or folded towel and place it between your thighs. Very gently breathe in through your nose. As you breathe out, feel your stomach muscles pulling down to the floor. Think of them pulling up and into your spine. Hold your breath and count to four. Squeeze the towel or cushion with your thighs. As you breathe in through your nose, feel your stomach gently expand into your fingers. As you breathe out, feel your stomach pull away from your fingers. Feel your lower abdominal muscles working. Repeat 10 times

Watchpoints

- Don't let your pelvis lift off the floor. This will 'shorten' the neck. Watch that your stomach doesn't 'bloat'. Instead, make sure that on the point of relaxation – when you breathe in – the stomach gently lifts. As you breathe out you should feel your stomach pull up and in, away from the pubic bone.

- Most people naturally want to breathe in and pull their stomach muscles in – this is a mistake. As you breathe in, you gently soften the muscles as they flow out into your fingers. As you breathe out the stomach pulls away from the fingers. Think of it as pulling 'up and in'. This will help you focus on your lower abdominals – strengthening and toning that area.

Working the lower abdominal muscles

Lie in the same position as in the previous exercise, knees bent. You can place your hands on your hipbones if you wish. This helps to stabilize your pelvis. Begin with the right leg. Keep your left leg completely still. Very gently breathe in and let your right knee open sideways. As you breathe out feel the resistance. Bring the leg back to the other one – breathing out and pulling your stomach in. Change legs. Now, breathing in, open the left leg to the side. Exhale and slowly close. Repeat 10 times, alternating legs each time.

Watchpoints
- Don't tilt the pelvis, and make sure that the supporting side is stable.
- Don't press your back into the mat.

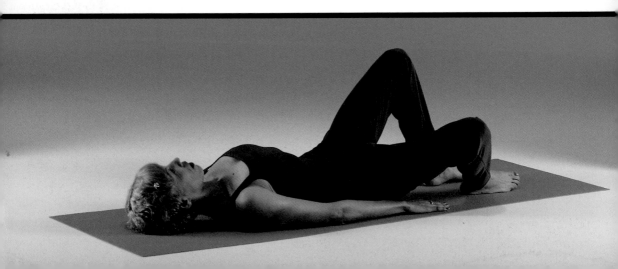

Working the lower abdominal muscles 2

This slightly harder version of the previous exercise is very straightforward. Interlace your hands behind your head. Keep them high up behind your skull and place the thumbs on either side of your spine.

Lift your elbows so that you can just see them out of the corner of your eye – without moving your head. When you can see your elbows peripherally you know that your arms are in the right place. Very gently exhale and 'float' your head and shoulders off the mat. Hold that position and repeat the movements of the previous exercise. Repeat the exercise 10 times, five times on each side.

Watchpoint

- As you lift your head, your focus shouldn't change – so you don't shorten your neck. If you shorten your neck you may tip your pelvis.

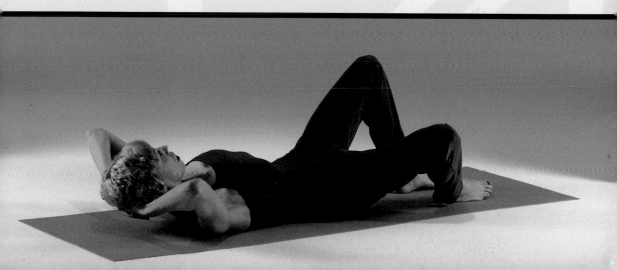

Basic abdominal curl

This exercise uses exactly the same position as the previous exercise, although the knee does not fan out. All the same rules apply. Interlace your hands behind your head. Keep them high up behind your skull and place the thumbs on either side of your spine.

Lift your elbows up where you can see them in your peripheral vision. Keep looking at the ceiling and gently breathe in through your nose. Relax the abdomen but do not 'bloat' it out. As you breathe out, gently lift your head and shoulders off the mat. Only go as high as you can. Do not strain your neck to hold that position. Breathe in as you go back down again.

Watchpoint

• As you breathe out, imagine that a piece of string is pulling you up from your pubic bone and under your rib cage. Pause until all the abdominal muscles go 'up and in', and flatten.

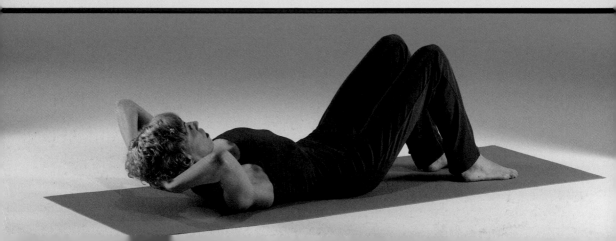

Single leg stretch

This stomach exercise is the first really coordinated exercise. It is a simple and basic exercise – which is not the same as saying it is easy.

Start in the same position as the previous exercise and interlace your hands behind your head. Lift your head and shoulders gently off the mat. As you breathe out, slide your right leg down, an inch off the floor. Breathe in, putting your head down and bringing your right leg back up. Breathe out, and slide your left leg down, an inch off the floor. Repeat 10 times, alternating the legs.

Watchpoints

- Many people make the mistake of exhaling before curling forward. If you do this, you will not get the same benefit. You exhale as you do the exercise.
- Keep looking at the same point on the ceiling. If you pull your chin into your chest you may strain your neck and won't get the results you want.

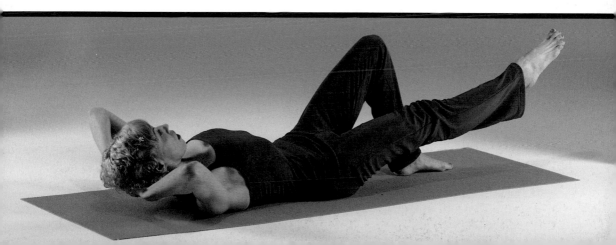

Basic sit-up

Lie on your back with your legs comfortably against a wall. Be close enough to, or far away enough from, the wall so that your tailbone is weighted to the mat. If your bottom is off the ground you're too close to the wall. Conversely, if you're too far away, you're legs won't feel supported.

Take your hands behind your head and lift your elbows to where you can see them in your peripheral vision. Keep the neck long.

Very gently breath in to prepare. As you breathe out, lift the head and shoulders off the mat, pulling your stomach towards your spine. Pause, breathe in and lower. As you breathe out and lift, the stomach pulls in, the pelvis does not lift. The neck is long, the head is cradled in the hands. You are not pulling your chin to your chest. Think of your breast bone and your head floating off the mat. Don't think of a sharp pulling movement.

Watchpoint

• The hands are interlaced high up behind the cranium and are not placed behind the neck.

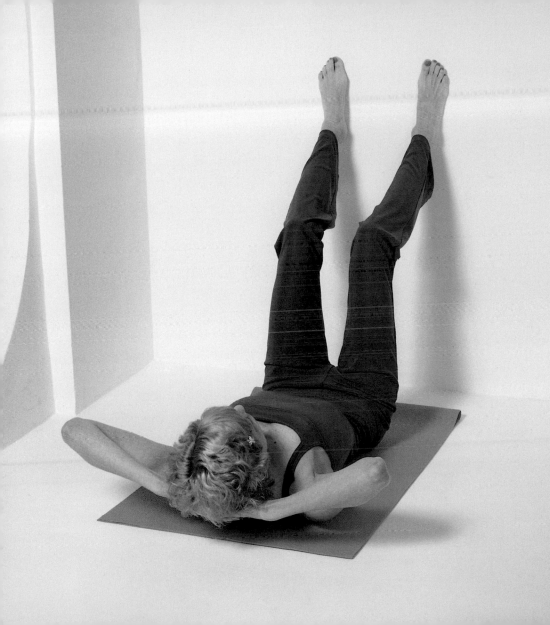

Sit-up with twist

This exercise is very similar to the previous one but with a 'twist'. Most twisting exercises work the oblique muscles at the sides of the waist. These muscles are essential for core stability and the mobility of the spine. If you want to have a strong stomach and strong back you must have core stability. If your muscles are too tight, you will have problems twisting and mobilizing your spine.

Remain in exactly the same position as in the previous exercise, breathe out and take a very small twist, easing the right elbow to the left knee. Don't get so high that you feel any strain in the neck. Breathe in as you release down. Exhale as you twist to the other side.

Watchpoints

- If you're unsure about this exercise, you can place one hand on the side you're working. As you breathe out, feel those waist muscles pulling away from your fingers. If they're pushing into your fingers, you've lifted too high. This may happen because your stomach muscles aren't strong enough or your back is too tight.

- With any of the abdominal exercises, it's important to lift only the head and shoulders as high as the point where your stomach flattens to your spine. If you lift too high and your stomach doesn't go in, you are building muscle. You might want to do this but you won't want to build muscle that will protrude. Perfect abdominal muscles are strong, firm and flat to the spine.

Advanced single leg stretch

This is the most difficult exercise in the programme. If you have any back injuries at all – don't do it until you feel strong enough.

Bend both knees into the chest and link your hands behind your head as before. Look at a point on the ceiling and breathe out. Let your head and shoulders 'float' off the ground.

Inhale. Exhale and stretch one leg out, pulling your stomach into the spine. Inhale and bring the leg back. Exhale and extend the other leg. Do five stretches on each leg. Only take the leg as low as the point where your back does not arch away from the floor.

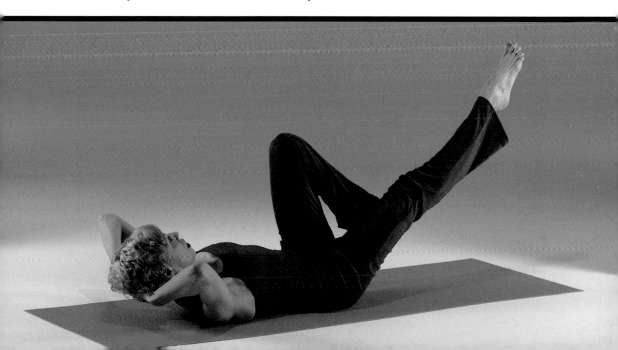

Side stretches and side lifts

The next three exercises are also for the abdomen but they are done lying on your side. These are called side stretches and side lifts. They are particularly good for the waist. The same rules apply as for all the abdominal exercises. It doesn't matter which side you lie on to start with. Do all the exercises in sets of 10.

Side stretch
Lie on your side, arm stretched out in line with your body, resting on the floor, palm down. Place your other hand on the floor in front of you, for balance. If your neck doesn't feel comfortable, place a folded towel between your ear and your shoulder.

Think of your ear 'lengthening' along the arm, so that you're looking directly ahead of you. The hips are stacked one directly over the other so that your pelvis is level, not tilted. It's very common to let the top hip rock forward. Glance down your body without moving your head. If you can't see your feet, they are too far behind you. If you feel any strain in your back, the first thing you should do is move your feet further forward.

Breathe in to prepare. Breathe out and lift your legs about four inches off the ground. Keep your feet gently flexed. You want to

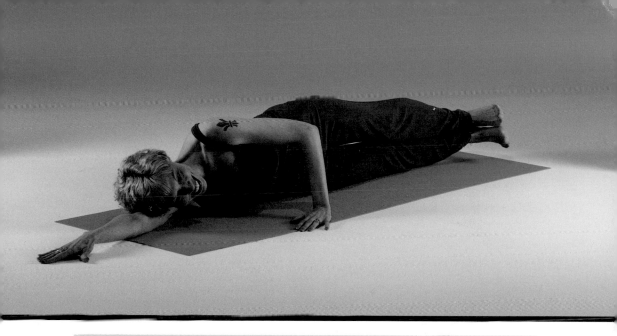

straighten the back of your legs. Feel the energy pushing through your heels as you lift. Breathe in as you lower. Do 10 on each side.

Watchpoints

- If you are unsure about this position, do it with your back against the wall. You can then feel how far your legs have to come forward to feel your middle back against the wall.

- Stretch your legs as far as you can without locking your knees. The knees are lengthened away, but slightly relaxed. If you're not sure about locking your knees or stretching your knees it's always better to have them slightly released.

Side stretch 2

The next exercise is simply a harder version of the one before – so all the same rules apply. Use a towel if you need to. Relax your top arm and shoulder. With flexed feet breathe out and lift both legs about four inches off the ground. Hold this position and breathe in. Breathe out and lift the top leg higher. Bring the leg back, breathe in, and slowly lower both legs to the ground and relax. Do 10 repetitions on each side.

Watchpoints

- It's really important for this exercise that you never allow one leg to become longer than the other. You don't want an imbalance in your pelvis.
- Correct breathing is vital. If you feel any strain in your back, try doing the exercise with your legs further forward.

Side lift

The next exercise is more difficult and you need to be reasonably fit to try it. Don't attempt it if you have any back injuries.

Lie on your side, with your elbow directly under your shoulder, your palm flat on the floor. Keep your legs in a straight line with your ankles crossed. It helps if can place your feet against a hard surface – e.g. a skirting board. This will give you a bit of resistance and help you get off the ground. All the same rules on alignment apply as in the side stretch. Keep your shoulder and elbow in line. As you breathe out, lift, pushing down through the supporting arm. The other arm lifts up to a right angle in line with the shoulder. Come back down again and relax. With this exercise begin by doing it four times on each side and slowly build up to 10. This will give you a strong, toned and, hopefully, very trim waist.

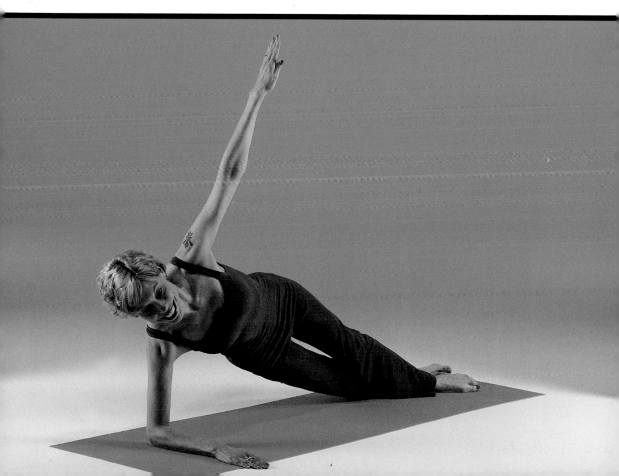

Back exercises

We now begin the back sequence. Back exercises are vital for a strong stomach and back because both sets of muscles support the torso. Without a strong back you don't have a strong body.

Cat stretch
A cat stretch is done on your hands and knees. Make a square of your body. Keep your hands under your shoulders, fingers facing forwards. Knees should be hip-width apart. Place your feet gently on the floor and don't lock your elbows at any point. As you breathe out, drop your chin to your chest and curl your stomach into the spine. Press your upper back to the ceiling, trying not to rock back and forth. As you breathe in, your tailbone lifts towards the ceiling, your chest presses to the floor and your head gently lifts. Breathe out and reverse the position. After 10 repetitions, relax your bottom onto your heels and just breathe.

  Watchpoints
• Don't lift your head too high or you may strain your neck.
• As you press your chest down to the floor (in the second part of the exercise), if you feel any pinching in your lower back you'll know you've gone too far.

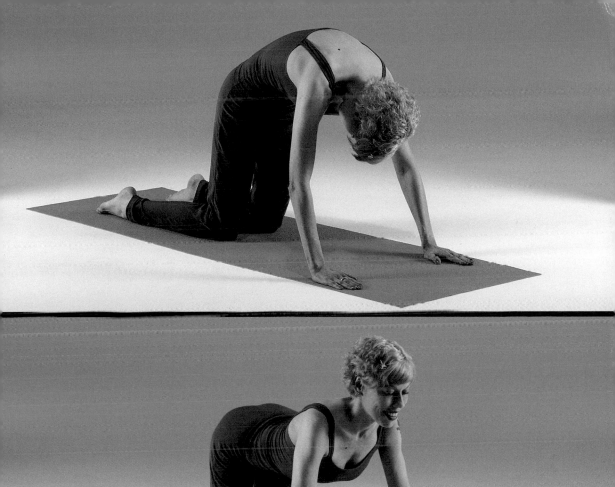

Back strengthening

Lie on your stomach with your feet relaxed. Your arms should be facing forwards and be just wider than your shoulders, which are relaxed. Keep your neck 'long' by looking down. Keep looking down as you gently press your hips and elbows into the floor and pull your stomach in. Gently, lift your head up (keep it independent of the body), focusing your eyes on the same point. Make sure you keep your feet on the floor. Breathe in, and gently come down. Feel your buttocks contract slightly. Do not contract them too much – otherwise you're using your buttock muscles and not the stomach. Engaging the abdominals helps to strengthen your back and lift your body.

As you breathe out and lift, imagine that the crown of your head is going forward towards the wall in front of you. Do not lift your head towards the ceiling. Ideally, you want as little pressure on the hands as possible. Relax your fingers and feel your shoulder blades releasing. Relax down again. Do 10 repetitions.

Watchpoints

- As you breathe out and lift, you should be able to get your fingers between your stomach and the floor.
- Whenever you do a back exercise, each time you breathe out, your stomach goes into the spine (just as in the earlier abdominal exercises). If you lift too high and you feel your back shortening, you've gone too far.

Back strengthening 2

This exercise is exactly the same as the previous one, except that this time, as you breathe out and lift, your hands 'float' off the ground.

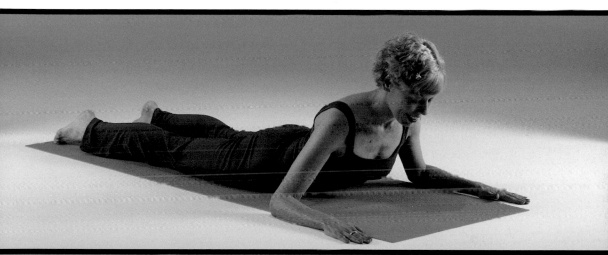

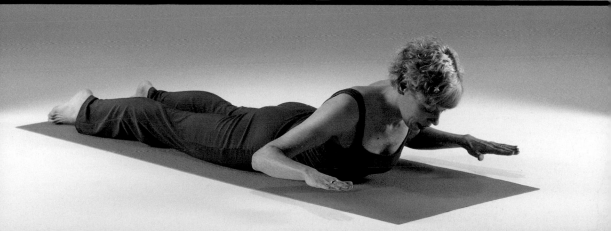

Alternate arm and leg stretch

This works your stomach and your back.

Lying on your stomach, imagine yourself in the shape of a rather small starfish. Your arms are slightly wider than your shoulders. Look down at the floor. Make sure your legs are comfortably apart and rotated slightly outwards. Exhale and let your left leg and right arm gently float off the ground. Feel your stomach doing all the work. Breathe in and lower. Exhale as you change sides. Make sure that as your stomach goes in your tailbone drops. Again, keep your legs straight and shoulders relaxed. Your arms and legs should be at the same height. Repeat 10 times, alternating between sides.

Watchpoint

• Don't shorten your neck, grip your bottom, or lift your arm and leg too high. Don't think of 'lifting' – 'lengthen' your arm and leg.

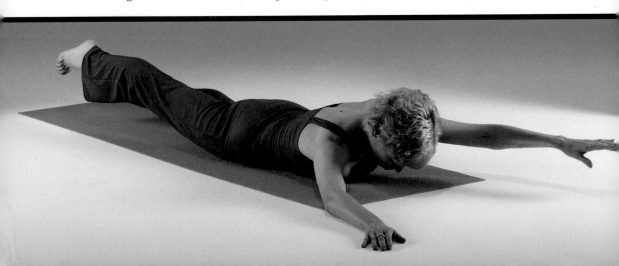

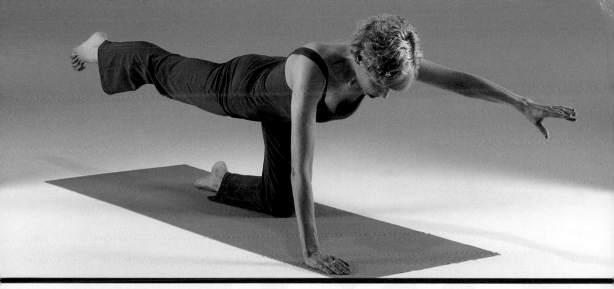

Kneeling arm and leg stretch

This exercise helps improve balance.

Assume the same position as the cat stretch (*page* 50). The spine is neutral and stomach gently in. Imagine someone's hand on your stomach. Breathe out, and let your right arm and left leg gently float away. Don't lift too high. To avoid this, position something like a kitchen roll across the base of your spine. If you lift too high, it will fall off. Keep your pelvis neutral, so that you don't tilt from side to side. Keep looking at the same point on the floor, so that you don't shorten your neck. Relax back into the starting position. Repeat, alternating arms and legs for 10 repetitions.

Watchpoint

- If this exercise feels too difficult at the onset, you can start by lifting one arm, or one leg only.

The swan – advanced back exercise

All the same rules apply as in the alternate arm and leg stretch (*page 54*). Once again, imagine you are a small starfish, lying on your front, with your arms and legs comfortably apart. As you breathe out, simultaneously lift both arms and both legs to the same height. Keep looking down throughout, and pull your stomach into your spine until you feel your tailbone drop.

Watchpoints

- Make sure that as your stomach goes in, your pelvis relaxes back; as you breathe, don't grip your bottom.
- Again, keep your legs straight. If you bend your knees the exercise won't be effective.
- Keep shoulders relaxed, stomach in, legs and arms straight. Your arms and legs should be at the same height.

Relaxation position – child's pose

Do this at the end of the back exercise sequence.

Sit back down on your heels with your arms close to your sides. Gently pull your head into your chest and curl yourself into a small 'ball' until your forehead touches the ground. Hold for a few seconds.

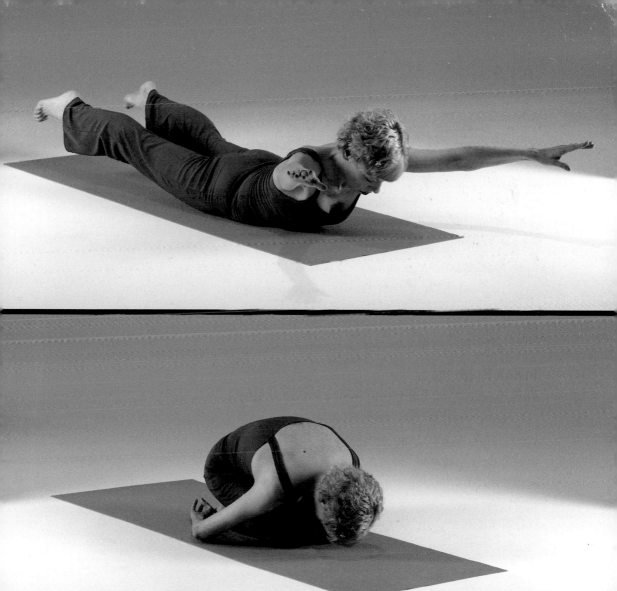

Legs

It is possible to create bulk by exercising the legs – if you do not do enough stretching. Everyone wants their leg muscles to be long, lean and lengthened as opposed to tight and bunched. There are certain parts of the legs, particularly the quadriceps muscles above the knees, that get bigger due to excessive use, while the inside thighs and hamstrings are usually undertoned.

The following exercises will help to strengthen, tone and condition your legs and help to make them more shapely. Any of the following exercises can be done with ankle weights. However, don't use anything heavier than one kilo. You want to tone and lengthen muscles, not build them up.

Inside thigh lift

This exercise will help tone flabby inside thighs.

You can do this lying on your side, either with your hand supporting your head, or with your arm completely flat. If you choose to keep your arm flat, it may feel more comfortable to put a towel between your arm and ear. Your top leg should be forward, in front of the body. If this feels awkward, place a pillow under your knee. The other hand is in front of you. The underneath leg (the one that is working) needs to be slightly forward, with your foot gently flexed. Again, don't lock your

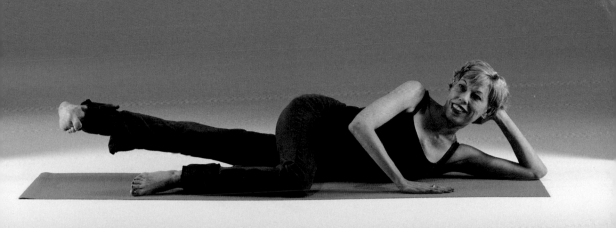

knee, but pull up the muscles, so that your leg is straight. If your legs are not straight, you'll be working your ankle and your foot much more than your inside thigh.

Breathe out, lift your leg and hold. Then slowly lower it. Don't lift your leg too high. Think of your leg going 'away', not up – as you want to lengthen and strengthen your muscles, not have them contracted and tight. As you lift and breathe out, your stomach pulls in, just like in the earlier stomach exercises. The energy is through the heel, working your inside thigh. Do 10 on each side.

Watchpoint

- It's important to remember that, in all the leg exercises, the instigator is your stomach. This means you should feel your abdominal muscles working. The same applies to all the upper body exercises.

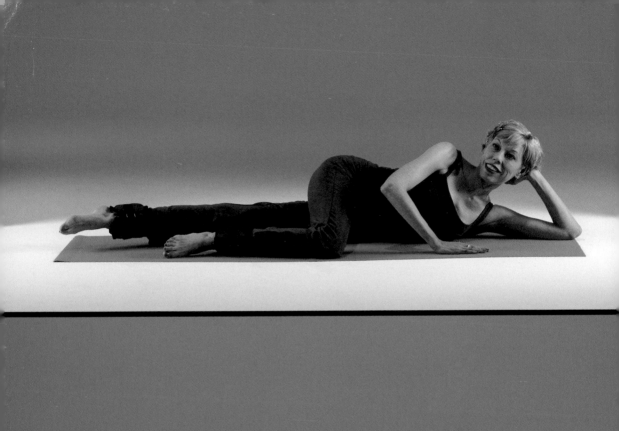
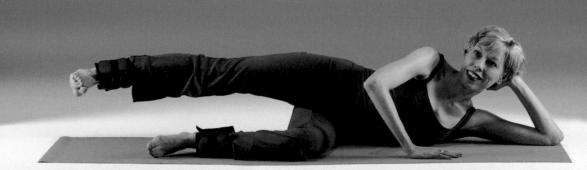

Inside thigh circles

Assume the same position as in the previous exercise. Gently point your foot. Breathe out and lift your leg. Slowly circle the leg in each direction. As you circle the leg, don't think of going up and down. Think of going out and away, so that you're almost touching the floor, as if you're circling around a coin. Do 10 little circles each way on each leg.

Watchpoint
• The knee is gently pulled up, the leg is reaching away, and you're circling down and away, not up.

Outer thigh lift

This exercise works the outer thighs and buttocks.

Take up the same position as before, only this time your underneath leg is bent comfortably in front of you. The top leg is straight, flexed and very slightly forward. If you've got any doubts about your back arching, you can lean against a wall.

The top leg should start the exercise at hip height. Very gently breathe out and lift the leg about six inches. Don't turn your toes towards the ceiling. Keep your foot facing forward, gently flexed. When you breathe out and lift, focus on the outer thigh and the back of the leg. Do 10 on each side.

Outer thighs and buttocks

Start this exercise in the same position as the outer thigh lift, but with both legs on the ground. Make sure your top heel is in line with your hip. Very gently breathe out and bring your leg forward, so that it's in line with the other knee. Breathe in, and lift. Breathe out, and lower and take the leg back. This is quite a demanding exercise, so start with five on each side, then gradually build up to 10.

Watchpoints

- As you breathe out, and pull your leg forward, don't swing it. Think of your leg as a 'resistance', so that it is the stomach that is bringing your leg forward, up, down and back, as you tone the back of the thigh. Keep it in line with the other knee. Your hip stays back, your stomach stays in.
- If you find you get cramp in your hip, this exercise might not be for you.

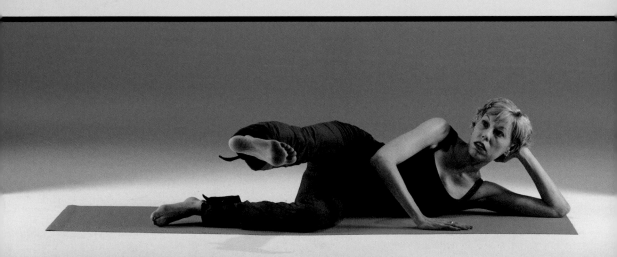

Outer thighs and buttocks 2

In the same position as the previous exercise, bend both knees, so that they are comfortably in front of you. Gently flex your feet. Lift the top leg, as if you're opening a fan. Then very gently breathe out, and squeeze the top leg to straight. As you breathe in, make a small bend in the knee. Breathe out and squeeze to straight. Remember – the emphasis is not on the bend, but on the squeeze. If you do a big bend, you'll be working your calves, not your bottom. Do 10 on each side.

Watchpoint

- If you get cramp, this indicates that your muscles are fatigued and it is best to stop.

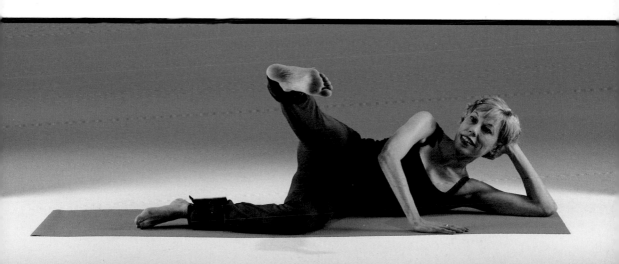

Hamstring toner and strengthener

Lie on your stomach, with your head relaxed on your hands. If you prefer, keep your arms at your sides. Do whichever feels more comfortable. Keep your shoulders relaxed. Very gently 'grip' your bottom. As you do so, you should feel your stomach going in and your tailbone drop. Inhaling, bend your right leg and flex your foot. Then gently exhale and straighten, keeping the buttocks squeezed at all times. Repeat 10 times then change legs. (The bend on this exercise is not important, it's just a preparation.)

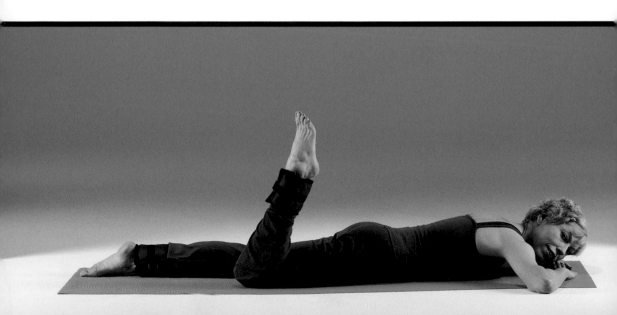

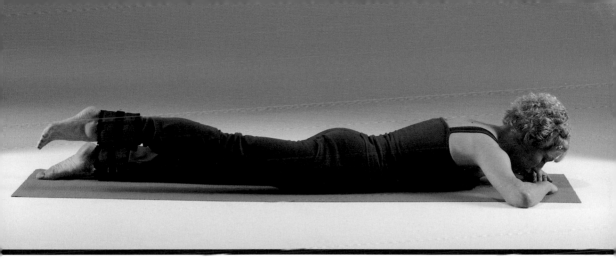

Bottom toner

Assume the same position as in the previous exercise. With a straight leg, hipbones down, stomach in, keeping foot relaxed, very gently breathe out and lift your leg up. Then slowly bring it down. This works the buttock muscles just under the cheek. Do 10 repetitions on each leg.

Bottom toner 2

This is exactly the same as above, except this time as you breathe out and lift, keep your foot softly flexed. Repeat 10 times on one leg and then the other.

Bottom toner 3

This is the last exercise in this sequence – and all the same rules apply as above. Starting in the same position, this time you bend your leg at the knee and flex your foot as you lift. Keep your hip down, and foot, knee and ankle in line, as you breathe out and slowly squeeze towards the ceiling. Repeat 10 times on one leg and then the other.

Leg stretches

It is vital that you do leg stretches after you've done any leg strengthening work. They are especially important if you have any back problems. If you've got a tight back, you may have tight legs. Sometimes it's difficult to know which comes first – a bad back and tight hamstrings, or tight hamstrings resulting in a bad back. Also, if you do have back problems you are likely to have a pelvic imbalance, which will mean that your pelvis is not in line. If you can get your body in line, you'll feel much more comfortable, and you will avoid a lot of problems.

Hold all stretches for 30 seconds.

Back and hip – gluteal stretch

Lie down on your back, cross your knees, hold onto your ankles, and very gently pull your heels into your bottom. Do this for 30 seconds with the right leg on top, then 30 seconds with the left leg on top. Repeat four times in total.

Watchpoints

- Don't let your bottom lift – it should stay 'weighted' to the ground.
- Don't hold onto your feet – hold onto your ankles.
- If it feels more comfortable, place a towel under your head.
- If you feel a strain in your back during this or the next exercise, then stop. This means you're working your legs too hard.

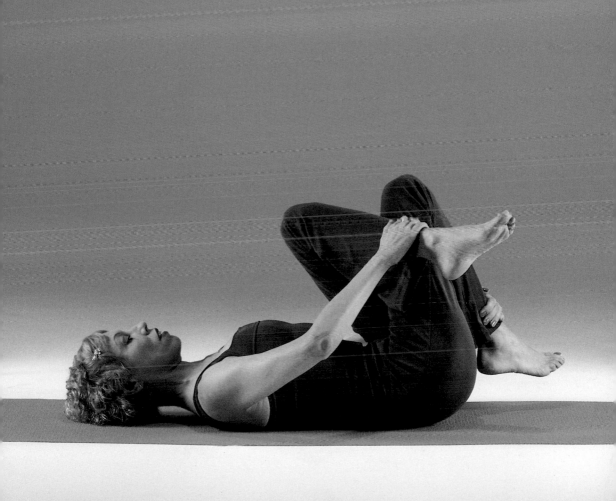

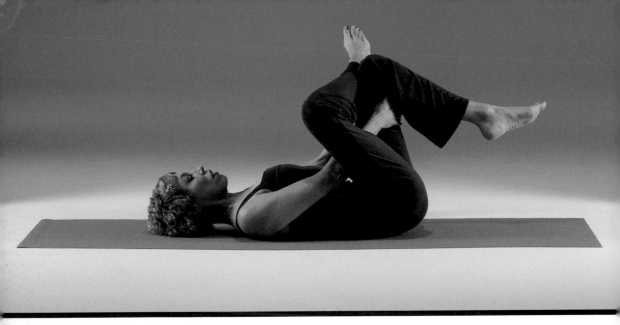

Back and hip – gluteal stretch 2

This is a slightly more advanced version of the previous exercise. It will help to release the hips.

 Lying on your back with your legs bent, very gently cross the right ankle over the left knee. Make sure it's the ankle, and not the toes. Gently, keeping your knee open, bend the leg into the chest and feel a stretch on the bent leg. Remember, on all the stretches, you should only feel a stretch on the working leg. Hold for 30 seconds, change legs and repeat four times.

Quadriceps stretch

This exercise stretches the large muscles running down the front of the upper leg.

Stand upright. Hold onto something if you feel you'll lose your balance. Lift one leg behind you, grasp the foot and gently stretch the front of your thigh. Keep your knees in line (check in a mirror if you're not certain). Ensure that your stomach is in, and your tailbone dropped. You should be stretching from the hip flexor all the way down the front of your thigh. Do not arch your back. Hold for 30 seconds. Repeat four times, alternating legs.

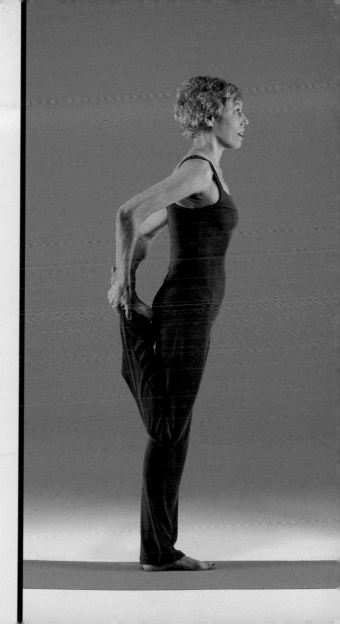

Quadriceps stretch (advanced)

Kneel down on your right leg. Extend the left leg so that the knee is directly over the ankle. Gently pull your stomach in. Lean back slightly without arching your back. Hold for 30 seconds. Repeat four times, alternating legs.

Watchpoint

- If this stretch causes pain in your knee or your back – stop.

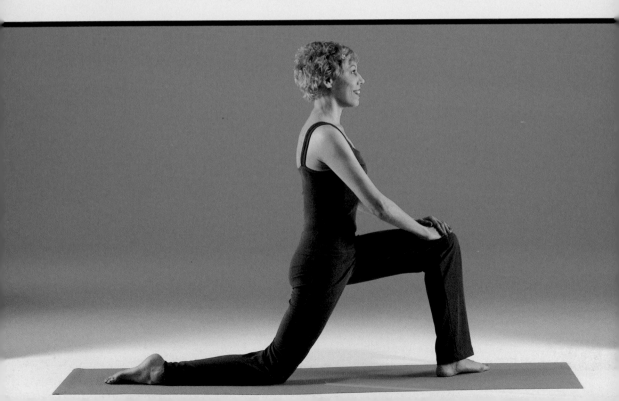

Lying calf stretch

Lying on your back, bend your knees into your chest. Place your hand behind the thigh of the leg that you're working, and stretch the leg towards the ceiling. Keep your foot flexed. Hold for 30 seconds. Repeat four times, alternating legs.

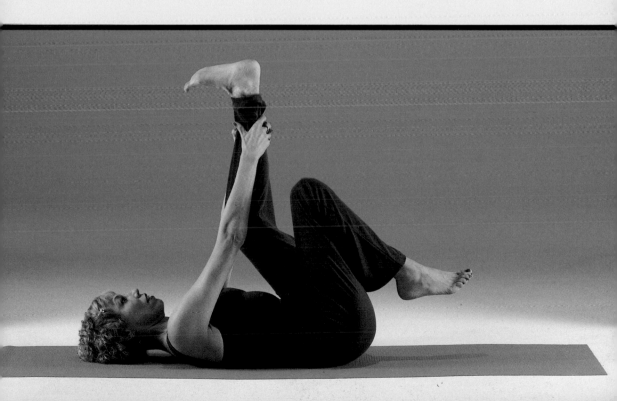

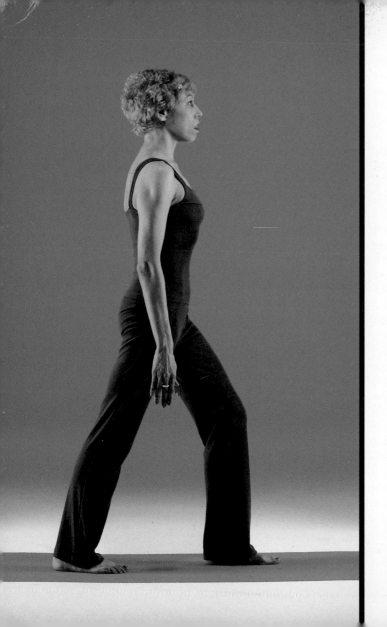

Standing calf stretch

Stand up straight. Take a step forward with your right leg, bend the knee slightly and feel the stretch down through the back leg. Keep your heel down on the back leg. Do not bounce. Hold for 30 seconds. Repeat four times, alternating legs.

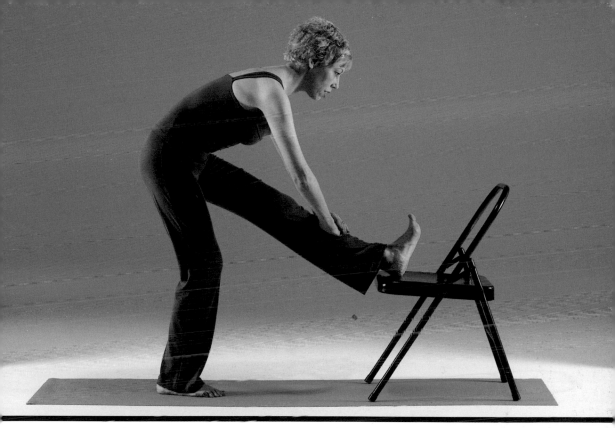

Standing hamstring stretch

Place your foot (gently flexed) on a chair and extend your leg. Keep the standing leg slightly bent and your stomach in. Neck and shoulders are relaxed. Hips are level. Slide your hands down towards your foot. You should feel the stretch in the muscle between the knee and the hip. Hold for 30 seconds. Repeat four times, alternating legs.

Lying hamstring stretch

Lie on the floor. Start with both feet on the floor. The arms are beside you and the pelvis is in the neutral position. Very gently bend your right knee into the chest. Grasp the back of your thigh with your left hand and the back of your calf with your right hand. Now gently unfold, straightening the leg with a flexed foot, and ease the leg towards you (as you become more flexible, you'll be able to place both hands on the lower leg). You'll know you're doing it wrong if your bottom lifts. If this is impossible, hold a towel around your calf and ease the leg towards you. Hold for 30 seconds. Repeat four times, alternating legs.

Inner thigh stretch

Sit on the floor with the soles of your feet together, stomach in. Hold onto both ankles. Gently drop your chin to your chest, relax your shoulders and let your knees drop to the sides. Hold for 30 seconds. Repeat four times. If this is difficult, sit on a cushion to begin with.

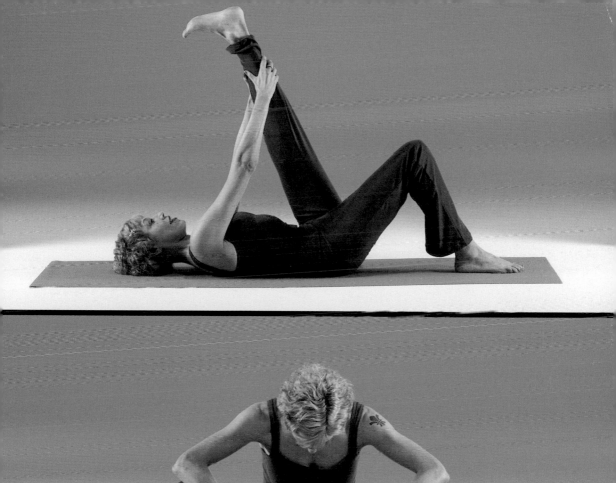

Advanced inner thigh stretch

Lie on your back, with your legs up a wall. Let your legs fan out to the sides as far as is comfortable. Make sure your stomach is in, and your tailbone dropped. If you feel any pain in your knees, stop. Hold for 30 seconds. Bring your legs back together. Repeat four times.

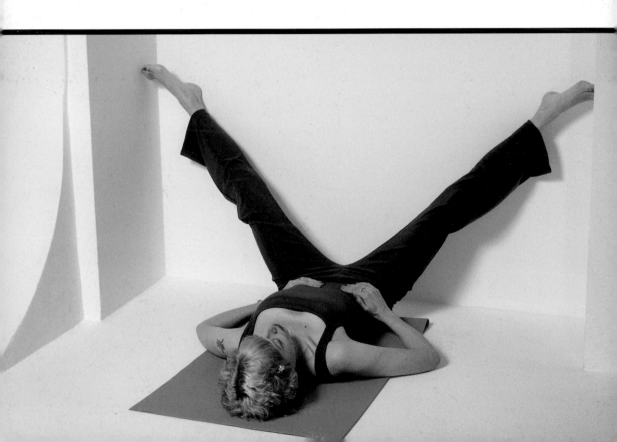

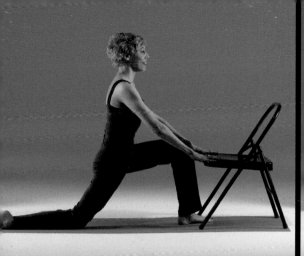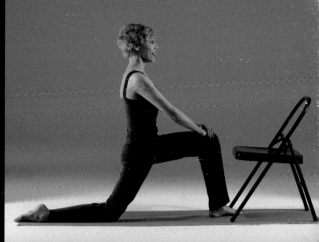

Hip flexor and front of thigh exercise

Kneel in front of a chair and place one foot in front of you with the knee bent. Hold onto the chair to stabilize your weight. The knee should be directly above the ankle and the toes should either be pointing directly forward or slightly outwards – whichever feels most comfortable.

Kneeling on the other leg, the foot behind you, very gently pull your stomach in. Press your hips forward and feel a stretch down the front of the thigh. Do not arch your back. Your stomach is pulled in and your shoulders are relaxed. Hold for 30 seconds. Repeat twice on each side, alternating legs. For a stronger stretch place your hands on your knee.

Watchpoint

• If you experience any knee pain at any time, stop. Pain in the knee is contraindicated in any exercise.

Upper body exercises

The following exercises will tone your arms, shoulders and chest. You can do second sets when your body builds up to it and follow them with the stretches, which are absolutely essential after upper body work. One combination is press-ups, dips and then repeat. An alternative would be a triceps press, biceps curl and then repeat.

Press-ups
This exercise is a slight variation of a press-up, which I use a great deal in my studio.

On your hands and knees make a square with the body. It is better not to kneel on a hard surface – use a towel or an exercise mat. To begin, knees are under the hips; the hands are under the shoulders. Cross one hand over the other. The neck is in line. There is no arching the back, the stomach is pulled in.

In this position, very gently, working with your entire body, tip yourself slightly forward over the arms. This does not mean you should arch your back. It is very natural, when assuming the press-up position, to allow your head to drop. However, try to keep the head in a natural position, neither forward nor back.

Begin by doing six repetitions with the right hand on top, then the left. Work up to a set of 10 or 12 with each hand on top. Very gently breathe in as you bend the arms, bringing the chest down. Breathe out as you push away.

If it is possible, do the press-ups in front of a mirror. When you press down, your head should not lower and your chin should not stick out. When you start this exercise you will feel your weight rocking slightly forwards and backwards. Try to stabilize the weight over the arms so that you get the most strengthening through the upper back, the shoulders and all the muscles in the arms.

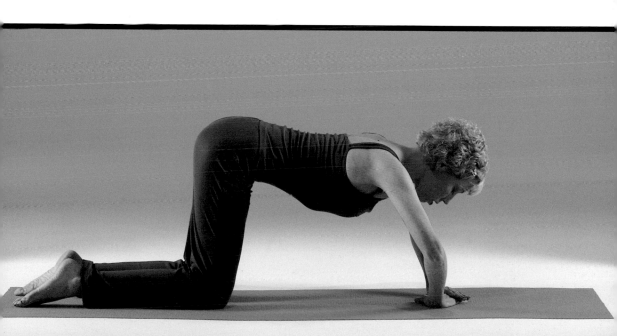

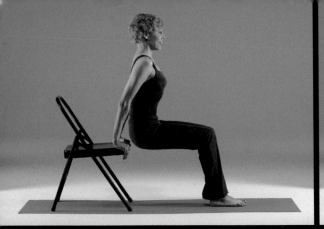
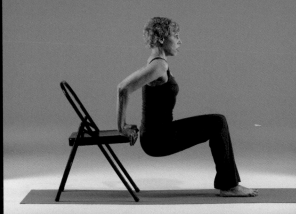

Dips

Most women find dips difficult to start with because of the lack of strength in the backs of their arms.

Using a chair placed against a wall for support, have your hands wide enough so that your shoulders don't feel pinched together. Fingers are facing forward. Make sure in this position that your knees are over your ankles. If they're not you'll be using your thighs as opposed to the backs of your arms.

As you breathe in, you bend; as you breathe out, you straighten. Make sure as you do the dips that you're sliding your bottom down the edge of the chair and that you're not sliding forward, as the body will automatically prefer to do, and taking the strain in the front of the thighs. You might only be able to start with eight repetitions – gently build up to 25.

Biceps curl

Holding a two-kilo
weight in each hand,
breathe in and bend
your arm up to
shoulder level. Breathe
out and straighten to
waist level. Try not to
rock as you do this.
Repeat 10–15 times
with alternate arms.

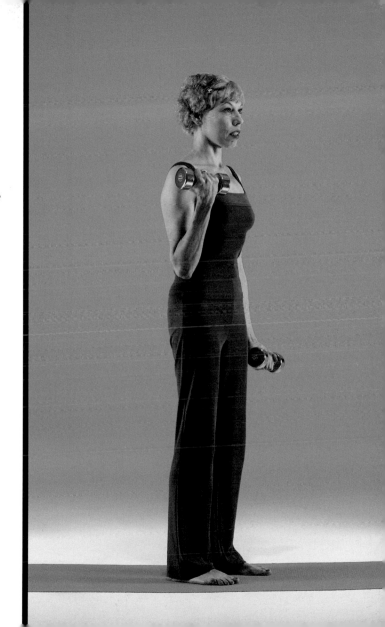

Triceps press

This exercise works the backs of the arms.

Using a firm chair, make a square with your body. Place your left hand and knee on the chair, keeping your right leg straight on the ground. Keep your neck in line with the rest of your body. Holding the hand weight, lift your right arm up as high as you can, keeping the elbow bent at a right angle, without twisting the body. Exhale as you straighten the arm behind you. Pause. Bend your arm back again. Repeat 10–15 times on each arm. You may do a second set.

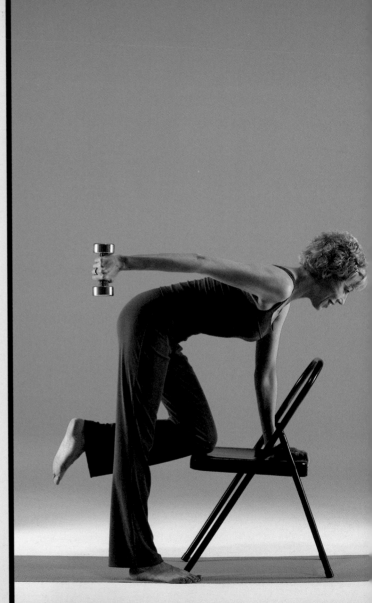

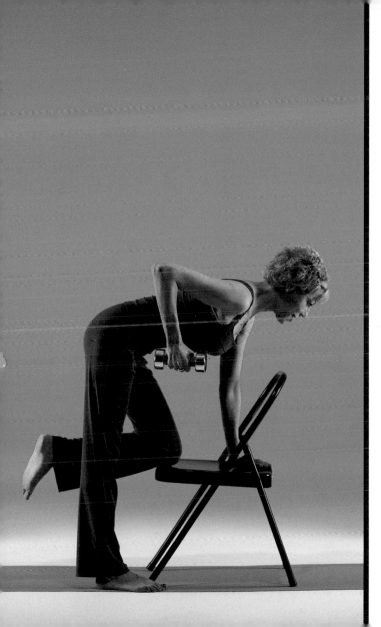

Lat exercise

This exercise works the latissimus dorsi muscles that run from below the shoulders down the back.

Assume the same position as in the previous exercise. (All the same rules apply.) This time you're using your arm to pull up and down. As you 'pull' – feel your lats doing all the work – imagine you're pulling up weeds. Pause. Repeat 10–15 times on each arm. You may do a second set.

Watchpoint

• Do not use your shoulders to do the work in this exercise.

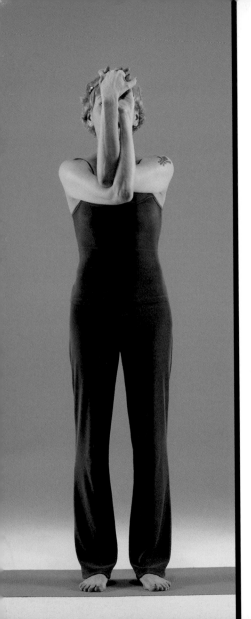

Shoulder stretch

This stretch can be done seated or standing. Cross one arm over the other and clasp your hands together. Gently push your elbows to the ceiling and feel your shoulders stretching. As you press your arms up, try to keep your shoulders down. Keep your elbows in line with your shoulders. Hold for 10 seconds and then relax. Repeat four times, alternating arms.

Watchpoint

- If you feel any cramp or discomfort in your shoulders or arms, you are not yet flexible enough to do this.

Arms opening

Lie on your back with your feet together, your knees bent and your thighs gently touching. The back should be in a neutral position, with no tension in the lower back. Place a towel under your head if it feels more comfortable.

Raise your arms above your chest. Imagine you're a tulip, and as you breathe out, your arms gently open. As you breathe in, bring your arms back together. Keep the curve in the elbows. Repeat 10 times, opening and closing.

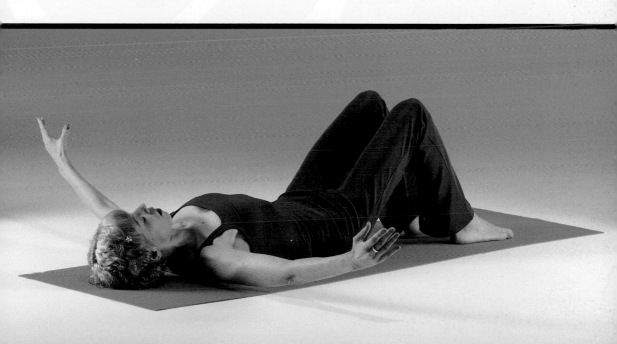

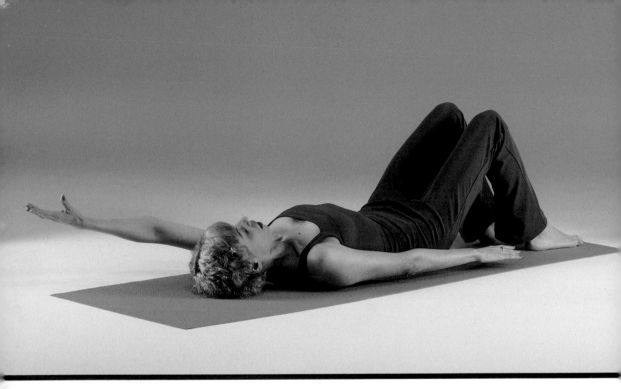

Backstroke

Start in the same position as in the previous exercise. Raise your arms and hold them out straight up above your chest, the palms facing the wall in front of you. Keep your shoulders relaxed. As you breathe out, simultaneously one arm goes down in front of you and one behind you. Breathe in as you reverse the arms. Imagine you're doing the backstroke. Repeat 20 times, 10 on each side.

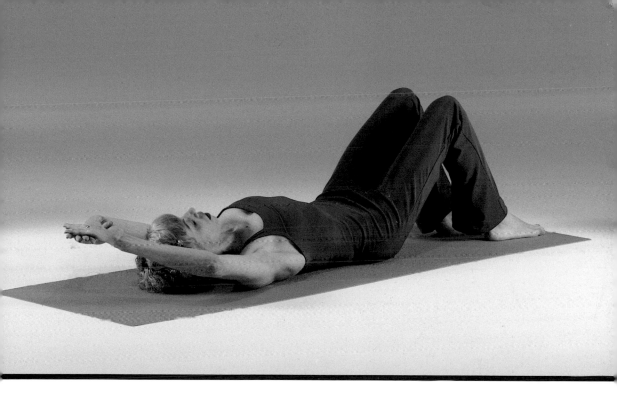

Lying shoulder stretch

Assume the same position as in the previous exercise. Place one hand gently over the other, so that you're making a diamond shape with your elbows. As you breathe out, take your arms as far back to the floor, past your ears, as you can without your back lifting. Repeat 10 times, alternating the hand on top.

Arm circles

Assume the same position as in the arms opening exercise (*page* 85). With your arms stretched up above you, breathe out and make a circle, so that your hands touch the floor all the way behind you. Bring your arms back and stretch towards your hips. Repeat 10 circles one way and 10 going the other.

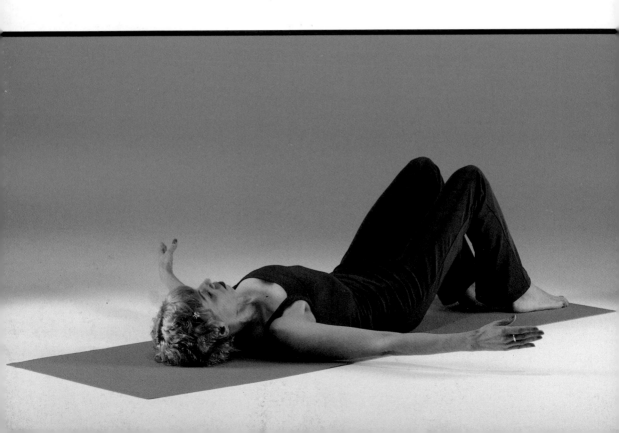

Rolling up and down the wall

This is a great way to relax at the end of any programme, but if you have any back pain don't do this.

Lean your back against a wall. Remember to always keep the knees bent, otherwise you risk straining your back.

Breathe out, and very slowly drop your chin to your chest. It helps if you count as you do this. Start to roll your back down, as gently as you can. By the time you get to a count of eight, your shoulders should roll off the wall. If your legs start to shake, bend your knees a bit more. Roll down as far as you feel comfortable and count for 10–20 seconds. Your arms should now be hanging loosely by your side like a puppet's. Gently move your head from side to side. Pause, and try to roll up, very slowly. Repeat four times (twice down, twice up).

Watchpoint
- If you've got low blood pressure don't do this, or you might feel faint.

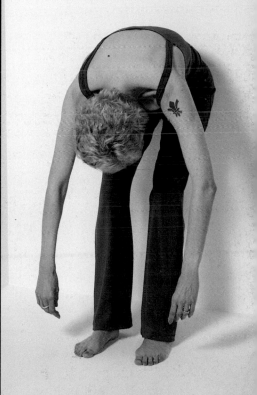

Conclusion

The benefits of embarking on this exercise programme are manifold. As in any DIY book, until you familiarize yourself with all the material and go through it at your own pace, it may seem a bit confusing. You will find that once you coordinate your movements with the correct breathing any apprehension will soon vanish.

While the material is still fresh, before you close this book, why not try a simple visualization exercise right now? Close your eyes – scan your body – visit each area. What do you feel? Is any area painful or weak? Do you immediately focus on one area? Try the postural exercises to get a feeling of alignment. Imagine how you wish to appear.

Your body represents the sum of its parts – therefore each part must be fully conversant with the others. Fluency can be achieved by allowing the mind–body–spirit connection to evolve. This is a challenge which can be met with calm determination and a vision of purpose. You now have the tools. Good luck!

For further information on The Body Maintenance Studio please send a stamped addressed envelope to:
Body Maintenance Studio, 2nd Floor, Pineapple, 7 Langley Street, London WC2H 9JA

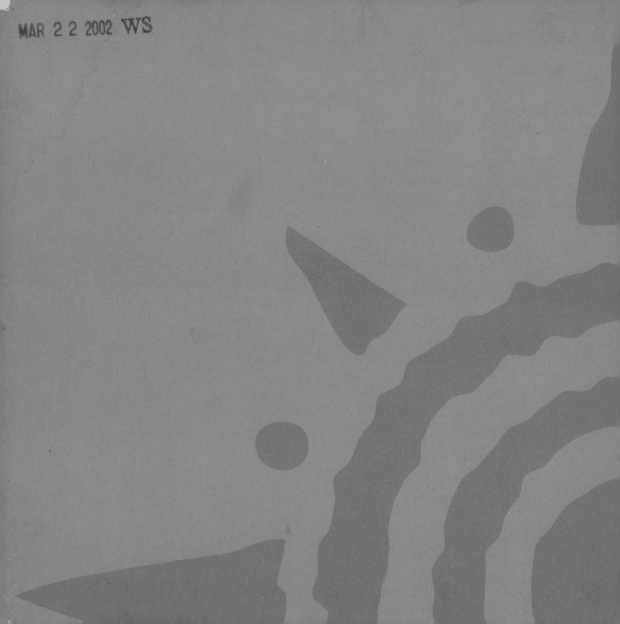